Mariana L. M. Aleixo
Jóice C. do Amaral
Raquel-Borges Poliana-Roma

Nursing care for diabetic patients

Mariana L. M. Aleixo
Jóice C. do Amaral
Raquel-Borges Poliana-Roma

Nursing care for diabetic patients

Case study of a resident of Cáceres - MT

ScienciaScripts

Imprint

Any brand names and product names mentioned in this book are subject to trademark, brand or patent protection and are trademarks or registered trademarks of their respective holders. The use of brand names, product names, common names, trade names, product descriptions etc. even without a particular marking in this work is in no way to be construed to mean that such names may be regarded as unrestricted in respect of trademark and brand protection legislation and could thus be used by anyone.

Cover image: www.ingimage.com

This book is a translation from the original published under ISBN 978-620-2-18313-0.

Publisher:
Sciencia Scripts
is a trademark of
Dodo Books Indian Ocean Ltd. and OmniScriptum S.R.L publishing group

120 High Road, East Finchley, London, N2 9ED, United Kingdom
Str. Armeneasca 28/1, office 1, Chisinau MD-2012, Republic of Moldova, Europe
Printed at: see last page
ISBN: 978-620-7-12062-8

NURSING CARE FOR DIABETIC PATIENTS

CASE STUDY OF A RESIDENT OF CACERES - MT

Enf-. **Mariana Lenina Menezes Aleixo** Enf-. **Joice Cristina do Amaral** Enf-. **Ma. Raquel Borges Silva** Enf-. **Ma. Poliana Roma Greve Nodari**

Summary

Introduction: Diabetes Mellitus is a heterogeneous group of metabolic disorders that have hyperglycemia in common, it has type I and type II, the latter being the most frequent form of the disease affecting 90% of all cases of Diabetes Mellitus. Men, in general, suffer more from severe and chronic illnesses than women, so measures focused on health education have been implemented to raise awareness about changing risk behaviors and the importance of self-care, in order to increase the life expectancy of this population. The participation of health professionals in caring for diabetic patients is essential. Nursing can articulate intervention actions by identifying the reality in which patients are inserted, using the Systematization of Nursing Care as a facilitating element in care planning. The aim of this research was to describe the behavioral habits of a patient with Type II Diabetes Mellitus, relating them to the nursing care provided in primary care. This was a qualitative case study, with structured and semi-structured interviews carried out between March and May 2016. It was concluded that the health-disease relationship depends on the behavior of the diabetic patient, and on the nursing care provided in a continuous and effective manner, which can both contribute to improving quality of life and prevent disease-related problems. In this context, this study has shown that the lack of adherence and knowledge about treatment, diet and problems hinders the whole process related to the health of this individual, which is confirmed in the literature studied and has shown the advantages of using the Systematization of Nursing Care Systematization of Nursing Care, since it provides a holistic view of the patient, enabling a plan of actions to be drawn up to improve the diabetic patient's state of health and minimize the onset of illness due to adherence to simple measures, which is only possible with early diagnosis and individualized and effective treatment.

Key words: Type II Diabetes Mellitus. Men's Health. Health-Disease Process. Diseases.

1 INTRODUCTION

Diabetes Mellitus (DM) is not just one disease, but a heterogeneous group of metabolic disorders that have in common hyperglycemia resulting from defects in the appetite and secretion of insulin or both (BRASIL 2016).

It is a chronic disease and affects approximately 8.9% of the Brazilian population aged between 30 and 69 (MOREIRA et al., 2013). It is a pathology that sets in silently and causes numerous complications for the body, causing symptoms such as excessive hunger, thirst, dry mouth, polyuria and weight loss (BRASIL, 2016).

DM can be classified as type I diabetes mellitus, type II diabetes mellitus and gestational diabetes. Type II DM is the most frequent form of the disease, affecting 90% of all DM cases (AMERICAN DIABETES ASSOCIATION, 2010). Excess weight, insulin resistance, dyslipidemia and systemic hypertension are frequent complications in DM II patients (BRASIL, 2013).

DM caused 4.9 million deaths worldwide in 2014 and 11% of total health expenditure in adults. In Brazil, this pathology was responsible for 28.7% of deaths per 100,000 inhabitants in 2013. Mortality from acute complications had a rate of 2.45 deaths per 100,000 inhabitants in 2010, of which 0.29 per 100,000 inhabitants were among those under 40 years of age (KLAFEK et al., 2014).

In general, men suffer more from severe and chronic diseases than women and have a higher mortality rate than women when the main causes of death are taken into account (CARVALHO and FERREIRA, 2009).

The realization that men have a shorter average lifespan than women started a mobilization in search of improvements in men's health, so health education measures were implemented to raise awareness of the importance of self-care, as measures to increase the life expectancy of this population with a reduction in potentially avoidable mortalities and a reduction in serious and chronic diseases (BRASIL, 2009).

According to Tavares et al. (2011), the participation of health professionals in caring for people with Diabetes Mellitus is fundamental. This assistance aims to prevent and treat the complications that arise as the disease progresses. Patients should be encouraged to adhere to and adapt to drug and non-drug treatment in order to lead a healthy life.

Nursing can articulate intervention actions by identifying the reality in which patients with DM are inserted, using the Systematization of Nursing Care (SNC) as a facilitating element in the planning of care appropriate to this population in order to propose a specific therapeutic regimen suitable for each individual.

Research is of fundamental importance for the construction of technical and scientific development in academic training, helping to identify aspects that interfere with the maintenance of health.

The aim of this study is to describe the behavioral habits of a patient with DM II, relating them to nursing care in primary care, using the SNC as a tool for nursing interventions, with the aim of improving acceptance of the diagnosis, adherence to treatment, reducing illnesses related to the disease, increasing the quality of life in relation to DM in the enrolled population.

2 THEORETICAL FRAMEWORK

Diabetes Mellitus

Diabetes Mellitus (DM) is a pathology that has a history dating back to the time of the papyrus, in 1872, in Egypt, the researcher Gerg Ebers discovered the first document referring to the symptoms of a disease characterized by frequent and abundant emission of urine, it is believed that the document dates from the year 1500 BC, but it wasn't until the 2nd century AD, in Greece, that the disease was given the name diabetes because it resembled the draining of water through a siphon, with the main symptoms - Polydipsia and Polyuria - compared to the entry and exit of water from the diabetic's body (TSCHIEDEL, 2006).

Doctors of various nationalities realized that the urine of diabetics attracted ants and that sugar levels could be related to the pathology, but it was two English researchers, Willis and Dopson, who carried out tests and confirmed this suspicion. The first ingested urine from a diabetic patient and said: "sweet as honey". The second heated the urine until it dried out and became sugary, and around 1650 Dopson discovered glucose, thus giving it the name Diabetes Mellitus (Mellitus in Latin means honey) (SMELTZER and BARE, 2015).

In January 1922, after tireless research, the first injection of insulin was administered, a milestone in the history of diabetes, used to this day as one of the main drugs in the treatment of the condition (TSCHIEDEL, 2006).

Diabetes is a chronic disease in which the body does not produce insulin or is unable to use the insulin it does produce properly. It acts silently in the body, so by the time the patient feels any symptoms, their body is probably already weakened and some organ is damaged (SMELTZER and BARE, 2015).

It is estimated that Brazil will rise from 8th place with a prevalence of 4.6% in 2000 to 6th place with 11.3% in 2030. In 2017 there were more than 13 million people living with diabetes, which represents 6.9% of the Brazilian population.

> According to data from VIGITEL 2016, in Brazil the frequency of adults who reported a previous medical diagnosis of diabetes ranged from 5.3% in Boa Vista to 10.4% in Rio de Janeiro. Among males, the highest frequencies were observed in Natal (9.8%), Curitiba (9.3%) and Belo Horizonte (9.1%), and the lowest in Boa Vista (3.9%), Rio Branco (4.9%) and Manaus (5.3%). Among women, the diagnosis of diabetes was more frequent in Rio de Janeiro (12.0%), São Paulo (11.1%) and Belo Horizonte (11.0%) and less frequent in Palmas and Manaus (5.8%) and Teresina (6.5%) (BRASIL, 2017).
>
> In all 27 cities, the frequency of previous medical diagnosis of diabetes was 8.9%, lower among men (7.8%) than among women (9.9%). In both sexes, diagnosis of the disease became more common with advancing age. This trend became more pronounced after the age of 45, and more than a quarter of individuals aged 65 or over reported a medical diagnosis of diabetes. In both sexes, the frequency of diabetes diagnosis was particularly high in individuals with up to eight years of schooling (BRASIL, 2017).

The disease can be classified into two types: Type I Diabetes Mellitus (DM) caused by the absence of insulin secretion; Type II Diabetes Mellitus (DM), caused by decreased sensitivity of target tissues to the metabolic effect of insulin, gestational diabetes and diabetes mellitus in association with other conditions or syndromes. Prediabetes is classified as impaired glucose tolerance (ITT) or impaired fasting glucose (FGL) and refers to a condition in which blood glucose levels are between normal values and those considered diagnostic for diabetes (GUYTON and HALL, 2011; SMELTZER and BARE, 2015).

Type I diabetes occurs mainly in adolescence and childhood and is associated with pancreatic destruction and consequent inability to produce insulin, caused by damage to the beta cells of the pancreas or by diseases that impair insulin production (GUYTON and HALL, 2011).

In type II diabetes, the pancreas produces insulin only in insufficient quantities to maintain normal glucose levels in the body. The main problems related to insulin in type II diabetes are insulin resistance and impaired insulin secretion (SMELTZER and BARE, 2015). With a reduction in insulin sensitivity, the use and storage of carbohydrates is impaired, increasing the level of glucose in the blood, thus stimulating an increase in insulin secretion in order to compensate for the excess glucose (GUYTON and HALL, 2011).

The most common form of Diabetes Mellitus (DM) II appears in approximately 90% of cases, affecting mainly individuals over the age of 30, with the exception of recent years when the number of cases has been gradually increasing among young people, as a result of obesity, one of the factors influencing the onset of the disease (GUYTON and HALL, 2011) resulting from a decrease in insulin sensitivity (insulin resistance) or a decrease in the amount of insulin secreted.

Insulin resistance can also lead to the development of metabolic syndrome, a constellation of symptoms including high blood pressure, hypercholesterolemia, abdominal obesity and other abnormalities (SMELTZER and BARE, 2015).

DM is one of the most prevalent Chronic Non-Communicable Diseases (CNCD) and among the causes responsible for the significant increase in the number of people with this disease are an ageing population, poor eating habits, sedentary lifestyles and obesity (BRASIL, 2014).

The first and main symptoms of Diabetes Mellitus (DM) are related to the "four P's": Polyuria, Polydipsia, Polyphagia and Unexplained weight loss. These symptoms can be present in both type I and type II DM.

In type I DM, these symptoms are acute and can progress to ketosis, dehydration and metabolic acidosis (BRASIL, 2014).

The onset of type 1 diabetes is possibly associated with sudden weight loss or nausea, vomiting or abdominal pain (SMELTZER and BARE, 2015).

In type II DM, the onset is insidious and the person often has no symptoms. The disease is often suspected due to the presence of a late complication, such as proteinuria, retinopathy, peripheral neuropathy, arteriosclerotic disease or repeated infections (BRASIL, 2014).

> Type II diabetes as a result of slowly (over years) progressive glucose intolerance, and as a result of long-term complications if diabetes is not diagnosed for many years (e.g. eye disease, peripheral neuropathy, peripheral vascular disease); complications possibly develop before diagnosis is established. Signs and symptoms of DKA, including abdominal pain, nausea, vomiting, hyperventilation and fruit-scented breath; untreated DKA possibly results in altered level of consciousness, coma and death (SMELTZER and BARE, 2015).

Early diagnosis leads to appropriate treatment, with a higher success rate in achieving glycemic control, which in turn has been proven to reduce microvascular complications in both type I and type II DM patients (MARASCHIN et al., 2010).

The diagnosis proposed by the Brazilian Diabetes Society (SBD) according to the 2015/2016 Guidelines, states that...

> in order to be characterized as diabetic, a patient must have symptoms of polyuria, polydipsia and weight loss plus casual blood glucose > 200 mg/dl, which is blood glucose taken at any time of the day, regardless of meal times, fasting blood glucose > 126 mg/dl. In the event of small rises in blood glucose, the diagnosis must be confirmed by repeating the test on another day, and blood glucose 2 hours after a 75g glucose overload > 200 mg/dl.

Fasting blood glucose is considered normal when the value is > 100 mg/dl. This criterion has not yet been made official by the World Health

Organization (WHO), but there is already a recommendation from the International Diabetes Federation (IDF) accepting the cut-off point of 100 mg/dl.

Impaired glucose tolerance occurs when, after an overload of 75g of glucose, the 2-hour blood glucose value is between 140 and 199mg/dl (BRASIL, 2015).

When patients are diagnosed with type II DM, they are given advice on how to change their lifestyle, such as health education, diet, physical activity and daily blood glucose monitoring, in order to avoid the various complications to which they are exposed.

The drug of choice is oral antidiabetics.

According to Brasil (2014), Metformin is indicated as a priority, especially in obese patients under the age of 65. An alternative is Acarbose or Pioglitazone, which can be considered for young patients at moderate/high risk of developing type II DM, provided they have no contraindications to the use of these drugs.

For people with type II DM, the recommendation is to combine diet and physical exercise in an attempt to reduce weight and reverse insulin resistance. If this is unsuccessful, drugs are administered to increase insulin sensitivity or stimulate increased insulin production by the pancreas. In some cases, exogenous insulin is used to regulate serum glucose (GUYTON and HALL, 2011).

For practical purposes, antidiabetics are classified into three categories: hypoglycemic agents, antihyperglycemic agents and those that increase insulin secretion in a glucose-dependent manner, as well as promoting glucagon suppression (BRASIL, 2014).

Risk factors are defined as characteristics or attributes whose presence increases the possibility of having a health condition. Risk factors can be classified as non-modifiable and modifiable or behavioral (SMELTZER and BARE, 2015). Among the former risk factors are gender, age and genetic inheritance and among the latter are smoking, poor diet, physical inactivity, excess weight and excessive alcohol use.

Among the main risk factors for Diabetes are: environmental risks, smoking, genetics, behavior, improper diet, physical inactivity, obesity and dyslipidemia (PETERMANN, et al., 2015). A sedentary lifestyle, alcohol consumption and an inadequate lifestyle are considered to be harmful factors that can trigger diabetes and/or other chronic diseases (SMELTZER and BARE, 2015).

In a study carried out in Cuiaba-MT, Ferreira and Ferreira (2009) described the epidemiological characteristics of 7,938 people with Diabetes Mellitus (DM) treated in the public health system between 2002 and 2006. The main cardiovascular risk factors identified were: overweight, sedentary lifestyle and cardiovascular family history. More than 80% of these people were also hypertensive. Acute myocardial infarction (AMI) was the most frequently observed complication.

If risk factors were controlled, 80% of cardiovascular diseases and diabetes and more than 40% of cancers would be avoided (BRASIL, 2014).

The natural history of the disease is marked by the appearance of chronic complications, generally classified as microvascular: Retinopathy, Nephropathy and Neuropathy and macrovascular: Coronary Artery Disease, Cerebrovascular Disease and Peripheral Vascular Disease (GUYTON and HALL, 2011). All of these are responsible for high rates of cardiovascular and renal morbidity and mortality, blindness, limb amputations and loss of function and a much higher quality of life than individuals without diabetes (BRASIL, 2014).

Pasqualoto et al. (2012), highlight other complications such as:

complications of metabolic origin, the determining factor of micro and macrovascular complications; Diabetic Gastroparesis (GPA); Diabetic Neuropathy (DN); Diabetic Retinopathy (DR), which is associated with 90% of cases of blindness in patients; skin and lower limb disorders; Diabetic Nephropathy (DN) and cardiovascular complications.

In order to avoid complications for diabetics, it is essential that there is prevention and that nursing professionals periodically monitor patients, giving them detailed guidance on the care to be taken in relation to glycemic control, adequate nutrition, physical exercise and especially with the feet, procedures which favor a healthier life (MASCARENHAS et al., 2011; MENDES, 2012; BRASIL, 2014).

All guidance should be passed on to family members or people responsible for caring for the individual with DM (SMELTZER and BARE, 2015). Encouraging self-care is very important for developing self-esteem and improving the patient's quality of life (BRASIL, 2014).

Systematization of nursing care for diabetic patients

In the history of nursing, the Nursing Process (NP), although it did not adopt these terms, began with Nightingale in 1859, passing through the transition from the empirical nursing care process to the transformations marked mainly by nursing records.

In Brazil, the EP was introduced by nurse Wanda de Aguiar Horta in the 1970s. The NP is the dynamic of systematized and interrelated actions, focused on the individual, their family and their biopsychosocial needs, which enables the organization of nursing care, in a holistic, humanized and ethical way, aimed at solving nursing problems (HORTA, 1979).

This activity is regulated by the Law on the Professional Practice of

Nursing and by COFEN Resolution 272/2002, repealed by Resolution 358/2009, which provides for the Systematization of Nursing Care and the implementation of the Nursing Process in public or private environments where professional nursing care takes place, and makes other provisions.

In the literature, we can find other names for the NP, such as nursing consultation, nursing care plan, among them the most used in recent years, the Systematization of Nursing Care (SAE) (HORTA, 1979, BRASIL, 2009).

Nursing Care is described as:

> (...) the private activity of the nurse, who uses scientific work methods and strategies to identify health/disease situations, supporting nursing care that can contribute to the promotion, prevention, recovery and rehabilitation of the health of the individual, family and community (...) (BRASIL, 2009).

According to Tannure and Pinheiro (2010), the Nursing Process is the method used to implement a nursing theory in professional practice. In this case, the theory used was Wanda Horta's "Basic Human Needs".

According to Horta (1979) and BRASIL, (2009), PE or SAE is organized into five interrelated, interdependent and recurring stages, as follows:

I - **Nursing data collection (or Nursing History**) - the purpose of this is to obtain information about the person, family or group of people and their responses at a given moment in the health and illness process. At this stage, the nurse carries out the nursing interview, collecting socio-economic data, family and personal history of illnesses, surgeries, medications and hospitalizations. A cephalo-caudal physical examination is also carried out, using propaedeutic methods such as inspection, palpation, percussion and auscultation to assess organ functions and the body as a whole. The patient's safety and privacy are paramount.

The nurse is able to identify the risk factors that make patients more vulnerable to diabetes complications during the nursing consultation, identifying them early on and intervening promptly, as well as establishing a bond with the patient and their family, helping with their needs, encouraging self-care, and helping with therapy and disease control, improving their state of health (SMELTZER and BARE, 2015).

From the survey of problems and demands for care, we identified and established the Nursing Diagnoses related to the patient's biopsychosocial dimensions (MASCARENHAS et al., 2011).

II - **Nursing Diagnosis** (ND) - the process of interpreting and grouping the data collected in the first stage and making decisions on the nursing diagnostic concepts that form the basis for selecting interventions to achieve the expected results. At this stage, nurses can work with two definitions of nursing diagnosis: the International Classification of Nursing Practice (ICNP) or the North American Nursing Diagnosis Association (NANDA). Nursing diagnoses are classified as real, risk, well-being and syndrome. They are composed of a title, defining characteristics and related factors.

> Based on the problems identified and the formulation of diagnoses appropriate to the patient's situation, it became necessary to plan nursing care that was appropriate to her individuality, so as to ensure that not only was the clinical situation overestimated, but that the biopsychosocial aspects took a privileged position in the nursing interventions implemented (MASCARENHAS et al., 2011).

III - **Nursing Planning** - determining the expected results and the nursing support or interventions that will be carried out in response to the responses of the person, family or human group at a given moment in the health and illness process, identified in the Nursing Diagnosis stage.

IV - **Implementation** - the support or interventions determined in the Nursing Planning stage are carried out. Support can be provided by both the nurse and the nursing team.

V - **Nursing Evaluation** - in this phase, the nurse evaluates the patient to determine whether the nursing support or interventions have achieved the expected result; and verifies the need for changes or adaptations in the stages of the Nursing Process.

According to Article 4 of Resolution 358/09 and, subject to the provisions of Law No. 7.498/1986 and Decree No. 94.406/1987, it is the nurse's exclusive responsibility to make a nursing diagnosis about the responses of the person, family or human group at a given moment in the health and illness process, as well as prescribing the nursing support or interventions to be carried out in response to these responses.

The implementation of the Nursing Process must be formally recorded, involving: a) a summary of the data collected on the person, family or group of people at a given moment in the health and illness process; b) the nursing diagnoses about the responses of the person, family or group of people at a given moment in the health and illness process; c) the nursing actions or interventions carried out in response to the nursing diagnoses identified; d) the results achieved as a result of the nursing actions or interventions carried out. All records must be signed and stamped by the nurse.

The Systematization of Nursing Care (SNC) is a reflexive and dynamic process. Its purpose is to guide nursing practice with quality care in a comprehensive and individualized way, totaling patient care, enabling the identification of problems, formulation of accurate nursing diagnoses, adequate planning and daily evaluation of the interventions carried out are essential for the recovery and rehabilitation of the subject (MASCARENHAS et al., 2011).

This activity requires nurses to have up-to-date cognitive and technical-scientific skills aimed at humanizing care in order to help diabetic patients achieve a better quality of life.

The experiences of Mascarenhas et al. (2011) allowed us to reflect on the implementation of the SNC, which requires nurses to integrate effectively with the multidisciplinary team, considering it an essential tool for the proper development of their actions.

> As alternatives to promote the effective adoption of the SNC, Mascarenhas proposes a closer relationship between the nursing team and the SNC, through knowledge and encouraging discussions about its implementation; overcoming technicality, which is still hegemonic in nursing care for individuals and, finally, the integration and practice of humanized and systematized care by the entire multidisciplinary team.

When dealing with patients with Diabetes Mellitus (DM), nurses must pay attention to intervention actions at all stages, whether in primary prevention with strategies aimed at avoiding exposure to risks, carried out by raising awareness of the risk factors for diabetes, such as sedentary lifestyles, obesity and unhealthy eating habits; secondary prevention through screening strategies with early diagnosis and the identification and treatment of individuals at high risk of developing DM; tertiary prevention through intervention against disabilities, and when this is no longer possible through recovery and rehabilitation (MENDES, 2012; BRASIL, 2014). The focus of nursing care should therefore be on the primary prevention of DM.

According to Malaman (2006), educational activities are of fundamental importance in the treatment of chronic diseases. It is the team's job not only to provide guidance on a disease that the individual will have to live with all their life, but also to help the user adapt their daily life and that of their family to the control of normal vital parameters.

Nursing has the main role of guiding people with diabetes in their self-care, looking for strategies and new ways to provide quality care, with simple interventions, such as help and guidance in glycemic control (MASCARENHAS et al., 2011).

These population-based interventions should be complemented by preventive support, developed at small group and individual level, in the micro space (MENDES, 2012).

One of the nurse's tools that shows favorable results is health education. It facilitates the nurse's involvement in activities related to diabetes control, brings professionals and patients closer together and helps form new concepts and practices that encourage patients to seek out more activities (GONQALVES and RAMOS, 2009).

The use of simple, clear and objective language by nurses is fundamental at all stages of treatment and in health education activities, which favors understanding about the disease, helping to adapt habits, use medication and participate in activities that help maintain health (BATISTA et al., 2014).

The nurse's contribution to the treatment of patients with DM is seen as favorable because it provides guidance and information on the necessary health care, as well as stimulating new habits, helping patients to live with the disease, improving their quality of life and expanding the possibilities of diabetes control.

The participation of nurses in the care of patients with Diabetes Mellitus, as well as that of the multi-professional team, is vital for restoring and/or maintaining the health of individuals with this pathology.

3 METHODOLOGY

Type of Study

This is a qualitative case study carried out with a patient with the chronic non-communicable disease Diabetes Mellitus in the municipality of Caceres-MT.

In the social sciences, qualitative research answers very specific questions and deals with a reality that cannot or should not be quantified. In other words, it works with the universe of meanings, motives, aspirations, beliefs, values and attitudes (MYNAYO, 2012).

A case study consists of an in-depth and exhaustive study of one or a few objects, in such a way as to allow a broad and detailed knowledge of them. Its results are generally open-ended, i.e. hypotheses rather than conclusions (GIL, 2008).

Population and study area

The data was collected in the municipality of Caceres-MT at the home of the patient with Diabetes Mellitus, using a structured questionnaire and a semi-structured questionnaire, between March and May 2016.

The city of Caceres is located in the Center-South mesoregion of the state of Mato Grosso - Brazil, bordering Bolivia, with a territorial area of 24,351.408 km^2 , hydrographic basin of the Paraguay River, with a population of 87,942 people, 44,098 of them men, according to the 2010 census, with an estimated 90,518 people in 2015 (CACERES, 2015).

According to the history on the IBGE website, the town of Sao Luiz de Caceres was founded on October 6, 1778, by dragoon lieutenant Antonio Pinto Rego e Carvalho by order of the fourth governor and capitao-general of the captaincy of Mato Grosso, Luiz de Albuquerque de Melo Pereira e Caceres.

The Municipal Health Department carries out the municipality's health policy in relation to medical care activities, promotes medical and dental care for the population; carries out studies of illnesses in the municipality with the aim of identifying the causes and taking the appropriate measures within the limits of its competence; cooperates with private institutions aimed at carrying out any activities concerning the health area (CACERES, 2015).

Data collection

Data collection began after the work was approved as a subproject of the study "Characterization of the National Policy for Comprehensive Attention to Men's Health and its relationship with men's health profile and knowledge about their health".

The interviewees were invited to take part in the study voluntarily. Before the questionnaire was administered, the Informed Consent Form (ICF) was read out and they were asked to sign it and enter their Individual Taxpayer Registration (CPF) number.

Two interviews were held in three meetings, one to collect specific data (Structured Questionnaire) and the other two recorded interviews (Semi-Structured Questionnaire).

The semi-structured interviews were conducted by the researcher face-to-face at the interviewees' homes between March and May 2016.

The instrument used to collect the data was a questionnaire made up of objective questions, which were answered orally by the researcher and the answers transcribed immediately. We also used a semi-structured questionnaire whose answers were recorded, with the interviewee's consent, on a *Galaxy S5 mini* cell phone and transcribed in the discussion.

The questionnaires made it possible to collect the necessary data to be discussed through the Systematization of Nursing Care, an instrument that contributed to the assessment of the individual as a whole, identifying problems and raising solutions pertinent to the needs of the individual studied, thus helping in the prevention and promotion of their health.

The structured and semi-structured questionnaires were adapted from the instruments used by Gil et. al (2008) in their study with diabetics in the city of Londrina-PR and Almeida (2012) in their study on the quality of life of diabetic patients in basic units in the municipality of Macapa-AP.

The individual's glycemic indices were checked during five (5) days of fasting and at random.

Study population

Participants were selected according to inclusion criteria:

1. Be male, between the ages of 20 and 59;
2. Having diabetes mellitus, whether or not they adhere to treatment;
3. Be a resident of the municipality of Caceres;
4. Agree to take part in the study and sign the Free and Informed Consent Form, after the researcher had given them a verbal explanation of the study's objectives and methodology.

Exclusion criteria were considered:

1. Under 20 years of age and over 59 years of age;
2. Be female;
3. Not adhering to the Free and Informed Consent Form;

4. Not informing the CPF number and/or not signing the Free and Informed Consent Form.

Data Analysis and Presentation

According to Minayo (2004), analysis searches for meaning in speech and support in order to arrive at an understanding or explanation that goes beyond what is described and analyzed.

The data collected was analyzed using the nurse assessment tool (SAE), with the help of assessment books such as: (NANDA, 2013; CARPENITO-MOYET and GARCEZ, 2011). They are presented descriptively.

Ethical aspects

This study was submitted to the Ethics Committee of the State University of Mato Grosso (UNEMAT), respecting the principles and guidelines of Resolution 466/2012 of the National Council for Health Research involving human beings, and is a subproject of the research project entitled: "Characterization of the National Policy for Comprehensive Care for Men's Health and its relationship with men's health profile and knowledge about their health" with opinion no. 686.372 of 11/06/2014.

The risk of embarrassment was minimal, as the identity of the interviewee was preserved while maintaining total anonymity.

4 DATA ANALYSIS AND DISCUSSION

History

R. B. S., 30 years old, black, male, complete high school education, salesman, married, Catholic, 81 kg, 1.65 cm tall, born in Caceres-MT, living with his wife and two daughters in the municipality of origin whose house is brick, has 5 rooms and access to basic sanitation, Medical Diagnosis of Type 2 Diabetes Mellitus.

He was diagnosed with diabetes more than a year ago, which was detected when he was hospitalized due to an abscess in his head. During laboratory tests, the pathology was found, which the patient said he already suspected because he had symptoms such as polyuria and polydipsia.

The patient reported using the medication as prescribed, but did not follow up with a doctor or the Family Health Strategy (ESF) team afterwards.

Family history: son of an unknown father, raised by a mother with diabetes mellitus and grandson of a grandmother with heart disease, who died of a stroke, and a grandmother with diabetes. He denies smoking, says he drinks alcohol three times a week, is allergic to insect bites, does physical activity twice a week, bathes twice a day and sleeps an average of 8 hours a night.

At the beginning of her diabetes diagnosis, she went on a diet to lose weight, as she was weighing 99 kg. However, she eats poorly. She only eats two meals a day, lunch and dinner. She mentions that she doesn't like to eat in between the main meals, sometimes she drinks pure coffee or eats a few water and salt cookies, she doesn't eat fruit and vegetables, she prefers rice, beans, meat and potatoes. She sometimes eats sweets, which she says she likes very much. He reports having a good relationship with his family, which helps him to control his daily habits. He works as a salesman in a building materials store with a family income of two minimum wages.

Physical examination: he was conscious, oriented, walking, cooperative, reluctant to change his lifestyle habits, reporting that he knows it's wrong, but continues to do so. Whole skin, no lesions, turgor preserved. Scalp and hair clean. Ocular cavity stained, pupils isochoric and photoreagent. Oral cavity with presence of all natural teeth, absence of halitosis, tongue with normal appearance. Cervical cavity with preserved tone and movements of rotation and flexion, absence of palpable ganglia. Pulmonary auscultation: physiological vesicular murmurs in the apices and bases of the lungs, respiratory rate was eupneic, good thoracic expansion bilaterally and symmetrical. Cardiac auscultation: performed in 10 foci (pulmonary, mitral or bicuspid, tricuspid, aortic, aorta, pulmonary artery, left atrium, left ventricle, right ventricle and right atrium) showed normal rhythmic heart sounds at two tempos (B1 and B2). Abdomen flaccid, hydroaerial noises present in the intestinal alps of the ascending and descending colons, bowel movements present daily. Light yellow diuresis present, Nicturia, Segundo
Information collected (SIC) 4 to 5 times a night. Genitalia not inspected, but no alterations reported. Upper and lower limbs (MMSS and MMII) with preserved muscle tone, movements of Abduction, Supination, Adduction, Pronation present, nails translucent, short and sanitized, superficial venous network visible, absence of edema, stains, lesions and peeling. SSVV: Tax: 36.7°C (Normothermic); RR: 20 irpm (Eupneic); HR: 84 bpm (Normocardic); BP: 120/80 mmHg (Normotensive); Fasting Glucose: 154 mg/dL.

Diabetes knowledge and living with the condition

According to Silva Junior et al. (2010), the majority of people with diabetes have regular knowledge of the disease. Ceolin and Biasi (2011) point out in their study that patients have essential information about the disease, which helps to maintain and prevent it.

[...]"... Well, about Diabetes, I know that it's a disease   related to a lot of, I guess, water in the blood. Eeee
(lol).... I have to control her..."[...]

For people with Diabetes Mellitus, knowledge of the disease is essential for maintaining and controlling metabolism. A survey carried out by Gil et al. (2008) in a university hospital in Paraná found that 80% of those interviewed had good knowledge of the disease. However, this "good" knowledge could become "excellent" with the help of the nursing team, who clarify the most frequent doubts and try to help these individuals to maintain and prevent health problems.

According to Rezende (2010), the importance of confirming that you "have" diabetes is obtained from the results of laboratory tests, a procedure that was observed in all the participants in his study: the patient needs proof to believe that they are diabetic.

[...]"... I found out when I was going through a health problem... then I ended up being hospitalized for 5 days, right? And the tests showed that I was diabetic..."[...]

Being diagnosed with diabetes requires a great deal of willpower on the part of the individual to follow the recommendations of the professionals involved in their care; acceptance is the first step for the patient to live in harmony with the disease.

[...]"...Well, actually, I was already suspicious, right? Sometimes I was just afraid to go to the doctor and have a test (lol) to confirm it... I started exercising again... I have diabetes..."[...]

The issue of acceptance was a problem, he says he "suspected", but the "fear" of being sure of the diagnosis meant he didn't seek help, which makes early diagnosis difficult, as the individual has a reaction of denial. Ferreira et al. (2013) state that the repercussions of the diagnosis mostly lead to a variety of responses that clash between acceptance and resistance. In their study, some of the interviewees accepted the decision to change their habits more calmly, while others resisted the necessary changes.

[...]"...eeee (lol), I know that it can cause me kidney problems... But I know I have to watch myself... in the future it could cause me greater harm, I know it could even cause impotence, right?"[...]

Diabetics have no idea what needs to be done to maintain their coexistence with the disease and that the lack of this can cause damage. Silva Junior et al. (2010) show that regardless of how long they have had the disease, patients are aware of the complications and say that the main ways to prevent them are through dietary measures, good information, medication, monitoring the disease through consultations and regular physical activity.

[...]".... Well, from the moment I found out that I'm diabetic, I've been

trying to change my habits, right? And... not just my diet, but the physical part, right? I'm trying to avoid sweets now, and I've started exercising again, which is sport, right? Which is soccer, which I try to do at least twice a week..."[...]

The issue of diet is always present in the speeches, and it is clear that there is a need for therapy focused on this issue, since making diabetic patients aware of the benefits of eating properly will have a positive impact on their quality of life, but the difficulty of accepting a balanced and restrictive diet is seen in this excerpt:

[...] "... Well, I know you eat a lot of fruit, right? Salads, vegetables. Just like that, right? It's something I don't usually follow very strictly, it's always lunch and dinner, I don't really like to have coffee in the morning, sometimes it's a glass of water, eeee (think a bit) about food in this case I had to go on a forced diet, right? Because I weighed 99 kilos, right? (lol)..."[...]

He also refers to the need to control his particular taste in sweets:

[...]"... sweets are something I particularly like, and at night, like I said, I'd sit in front of the TV with a cold can of moga milk and go away..."[...]

The difficulty in following an adequate diet is related to the habits acquired, the set schedule, the cultural value of the food, the socio-economic conditions and the psychological issue involved. Transgression and food cravings are always present in the daily life of diabetics (PERES et al., 2007). The need to change habits was perceived as an essential part of treatment by the majority of participants in the study carried out by Pontieri and Bachion (2010), who noted that it is difficult to do so, as sometimes the person's type of work can be a barrier to eating more properly.

[...]"...Especially at lunchtime, I used to go to the store for lunch sometimes, right? And I'd finish lunch and it used to be a habit to go to the grocery store and eat two of those 0.50 cent sweets there (lol), nowadays that's something I haven't done for a long time..."[...]

Alcoholism is one of the most alarming conditions in this case. We didn't find many studies reporting on alcohol abuse by diabetic patients, which is due to the fact that most studies are carried out with people over the age of 50 who, for the most part, don't use alcohol because they have other associated pathologies, which make frequent use difficult.

[...]... "I know I can't drink alcohol, right? But it's something I like to do.... I like to drink my beer, right? So, especially on Fridays, Saturdays, sometimes people do something on Sundays, right? rsrsrs....ai always end up impending, right?"...[...]

The Brazilian Diabetes Society (2015) recommends limiting alcohol intake in diabetic patients to one dose or less for women and two doses or less for men, an average equivalent of 15g of ethanol. Excessive alcohol intake can mask symptoms such as hypoglycemia, reduce hepatic glucose production and increase the production of ketone bodies.

[...]..." When I found out I had diabetes, my doctor told me to go to a nutritionist, right? So that I could see what I could be eating, so that I could control my diet, right? And so I didn't go to the doctor again, I just followed his advice about taking my medication...[...]"

What makes it difficult to maintain health in this case is the fact that the patient lives in an area not covered by the Family Health Strategy (ESF). The lack of a multi-professional team to assist this individual and collaborate in maintaining and controlling his health is essential.

In Brazil, the study carried out by Ferreira and Ferreira (2009) in Cuiaba/MT described the epidemiological characteristics of 7,938 people with diabetes treated in the public health system between 2002 and 2006. The main cardiovascular risk factors identified were: overweight, sedentary lifestyle and cardiovascular family history. More than 80% of these people were also diagnosed with hypertension. Acute Myocardial Infarction (AMI) was the most frequently observed complication. Another important result was the finding that when patients arrive at the Basic Health Unit (BHU), they already show signs of advanced stages of the disease, which demonstrates, among other factors, the difficulties of early diagnosis and the implementation of prevention measures.

Nursing diagnoses and care

Ineffective control of the therapeutic regimen related to insufficient knowledge

- Recognize what the patient knows about their condition;
- Provide the patient with information about their medical condition;
- Provide time and space for patients to express their feelings, doubts and concerns;

- Check for family and other factors that hinder the patient's growth and adherence to treatment;

- Promote confidence and positive self-efficacy by using success stories from other patients;
- Reducing anxiety, developing trust, providing correct and relevant information, among others;
- Promote patient and family learning by explaining the disease process, treatment regimen, side effects, signs and symptoms of complications, etc.
- Describe the reasons behind the control/therapy/treatment recommendations.

Risk of unstable blood glucose related to unbalanced food intake

- Helping patients to maintain adequate blood glucose levels as a way of improving their quality of life;
- Guide the patient and close family members on diabetes treatment, including the use of insulin and/or oral agents, monitoring fluid intake, carbohydrate replacement and when to seek professional help;
  - Restrict foods and drinks high in sugar;
- Plan a balanced diet rich in vitamins and nutrients to stabilize the glycemic level;
- Advise the patient on the intervals between meals, avoiding long intervals between meals;
  - Encourage self-monitoring of blood glucose levels.

Sedentary lifestyle related to poor knowledge of the health benefits of physical activity, as evidenced by verbal reports

- Discuss the benefits of exercise, such as reduced calorie absorption, preservation of lean muscle mass, reduced appetite, increased oxygen absorption, improved self-esteem and restorative sleep, increased calorie expenditure, maintenance of weight loss, among others;

- Help the patient identify a realistic exercise program that is in line with their reality and that they can follow in their routine, taking into account their personal preferences, lifestyle and physical limitations;
- Discuss the aspects of starting the exercise program, starting gradually and easily, setting a daily walking program, consulting a physical trainer, stopping immediately if any discomfort occurs, such as chest pain or dizziness, dyspnea, vertigo, nausea and loss of control and muscle tone;
- Encourage the patient to increase interest and motivation by developing contact with lists of realistic short- and long-term goals, keeping the patient in touch with others who practice the same physical activity.

Ineffective self-control of health related to the complexity of the therapeutic regimen evidenced by difficulty in following the proposed guidelines

- To investigate the factors that contribute to and cause non-adherence to the therapeutic regimen;
- Make patients aware of the components that balance glycemic levels and the benefits of physical activity;
    - Encourage the patient to follow a weight control program;
    - Help the patient anticipate environmental considerations;
- Advise the patient to maintain a routine regarding food intake and exercise;
- Familiarize the patient with acceptable glycemic levels and signs and symptoms that can trigger crises and/or serious alterations;
    - Teaching the basics of balanced nutritional intake;
    - To warn about the risks of obesity;

- Help patients maintain their weight throughout their lives.

Unbalanced nutrition: more than the body needs related to excessive intake in relation to metabolic needs, evidenced by overweight

- Discuss the need to reduce your calorie intake and limit your intake of fats and sugars;
    - Instruct and help with food selection;
    - Encourage the patient to lose weight;
- Encourage the patient to maintain a feeding routine, including "when" and "where" the food is eaten and the circumstances and feelings surrounding the food intake.

Impaired sleep pattern related to Nicturia evidenced by verbal report

- Encourage the use of prescribed medication;
- Advise the patient on the limit of liquids ingested during the night;
- Limit liquids to two to three hours before bedtime, as recommended.

Lifestyle-related self-neglect evidenced by verbal report

- Hold the patient responsible for their own behavior;
- Discuss with the patient the extent of their responsibility for their current state of health;
- Determine whether the patient has appropriate knowledge about the condition of health care;

- Encourage the patient to take as much responsibility for self-care as possible;
- Discuss the consequences of not dealing with your own responsibilities in maintaining your health;
    - Design a behavior change program;
    - Reinforce constructive decisions about health needs.

Anxiety related to the change in health status evidenced by having Diabetes Mellitus

- Offering real information on diagnosis, treatment and prognosis;
- Try to understand the patient's perspective on the feared situation;
    - Listen carefully to the patient;
    - Encourage the expression of feelings, perceptions and fears;
    - Identify changes in anxiety levels;
    - Guiding the patient in the use of relaxation techniques.

Medication care

Glibenclamide 5mg Oral

- Take the medication as recommended and do not interrupt treatment without the doctor's knowledge;
- Inform the patient of the most frequent adverse reactions related to the use of the medication and that, in the event of any of them occurring, especially those that are uncommon and uncontrollable, the doctor should be informed;

- Educate the patient about the disease, the importance of following the recommended therapeutic and dietary regimen, the signs and symptoms of hyperglycemia (polydipsia, sialorrhea, xeroderma and frequent diuresis) and hypoglycemia (polyphagia, sweating, tremor, agitation, irritability, headache, sleep disorders, mood swings and transient neurological disorders, changes in speech or vision and a feeling of paralysis and measures to prevent infections). Medication is not a substitute for dietary restrictions. When possible, recommend that the client be accompanied by a nutritionist;

- May cause hypoglycemia. Recommend that the patient control their blood glucose using a device that checks the glycemic value.

• May cause vertigo. It is recommended that patients avoid driving and other activities that require alertness when using this medication and/or experiencing this symptom;

• Oral route: the tablets should not be chewed, they should be swallowed whole with a little liquid; the first dose should be taken after the first substantial meal (ANVISA, 2014).

Metformin 850mg Oral

• Instruct the patient to take the medication as recommended and not to stop treatment without the doctor's knowledge, even if they show improvement;

• Inform the patient of the most frequent adverse reactions related to the use of the medication, and if any of these occur, the doctor should be notified immediately;

• Please note that the medication may cause a metallic taste;

• Recommend that clients avoid driving or performing activities that require alertness if they are experiencing symptoms of vertigo and/or drowsiness;

- In the event of reactions such as difficulty breathing, weakness, muscle pain, drowsiness or sudden Gastrointestinal (GI) discomfort, discontinue use of the medication and notify your doctor immediately.

- Oral route: the medication should be administered with food to avoid GI upsets (ANVISA, 2014).

Quality nursing care plays a fundamental role in the day-to-day life of this patient, who is of childbearing age and suffering from a chronic illness, since nurses have the tools to help plan care, with a view to promoting and preventing health, thus avoiding the problems inherent in the illness.

Nurses from the Family Health Strategies, in primary care, with their promotion, prevention and protection actions, help to maintain the health of individuals, and if they have a chronic disease, such as Diabetes Mellitus, the nurse and the multi-professional team can minimize the problems caused by the pathology, Given that from the moment the patient is diagnosed with a disease that has no cure, there are expectations about the disease, doubts about living with it and adherence to treatment, the correct intervention and a look beyond the pathology reduces the disorders in relation to the disease and helps in the daily life of this individual.

5 FINAL CONSIDERATIONS

The health-disease relationship depends on the behavior of the diabetic patient, and on the nursing care provided in a continuous and effective manner, which can both contribute to improving quality of life and prevent disease-related problems.

In this context, this study has shown that the lack of adherence and knowledge about treatment, diet and problems makes it difficult to maintain the health of patients with diabetes mellitus. This is confirmed in the literature studied and the advantages of using the Systematization of Nursing Care have been proven, since it enables a holistic view of the patient, favoring the development of a plan of actions that improve the state of health of the diabetic patient and minimize the appearance of problems due to adherence to simple measures, which is only possible with early diagnosis and individualized and effective treatment.

In view of the situation presented, there is a need for integrated care between the hospital network and primary care, i.e. an effective referral and counter-referral service that enables continuous monitoring and comprehensive care for patients with diabetes, which involves a multi-professional health team so that the treatment is really effective and the therapeutic regimen prescribed by these professionals provides healthy lifestyle habits that will reflect positively on the quality of life of patients with diabetes.

This case study made it possible to identify the risk factors inherent in the pathology of this patient, who is male, young, black, with a chronic illness, and the most appropriate way of dealing with this type of vulnerable and under-served public.

This confirms that there is a need for studies addressing the experiences of diabetics, as seen by Rezende (2010), in municipal Basic Health Units, and a reflection on this pathology involving more municipalities, which would bring current data to the municipal level and facilitate decision-making by managers to improve and/or build new public policies aimed at this public.

In this sense, this research has made a qualitative contribution at the level of the municipality studied, with this data being used as support material for health education for the population, and helping the academic population to identify the necessary interventions to be carried out in order to improve the living conditions and health of this public.

BIBLIOGRAPHICAL REFERENCES

ALMEIDA, A. N. F. **Quality of life of patients with Diabetes Mellitus:** comparative study of two assistance programs of the basic health unit of the Federal University of Amapa, in the municipality of Macapa, Amapa, 2012. Dissertation (master's degree). Fundapao Universidade Federal do Amapa, Postgraduate Program in Health Sciences. Macapa, 2012.

American Diabetes association. **Diagnosis and classification of diabetes mellitus.** Diabetes Care. 2010. Accessed on 20/12/2015.

ANVISA. National Health Surveillance Agency. **Model package leaflet, Glibenclamide 5mg and Metformin 850mg.** Brasilia, 2014. Available at: <http://www.anvisa.gov.br/datavisa/fila-bula/frmVisualizarBula>. Accessed on: 20/05/2017.

BATISTA, M. G.; MELO, R. K. A.; MAXIMIANO, D. A. F. M.; SILVA, P. E.; LUCENA, A. L. R.; VIEIRA, K. F. L. Diabetes Mellitus: characteristics of nursing assistance and care for the elderly. **Revista de Enfermagem UFPE** online. Recife, Dec. 2014. Available at: <www.revista.ufpe.br/revistaenfermagem/index.php/revista/article/download/1 0992>. Accessed on: 25/07/2016.

BRAZIL. Ministry of Health. Secretariat of Health Care. Department of Primary Care. **Strategies for the care of people with chronic diseases:** Diabetes Mellitus. Ministerio da Saude, Secretaria de Atenpao a Saude, Departamento de Atenpao Basica. Brasilia: Ministry of Health, 2014.

BRAZIL. Ministry of Health. Health Surveillance Secretariat. Department of Surveillance of Non-Communicable Diseases and Health Promotion. **Vigitel Brazil 2016:** surveillance of risk and protective factors for chronic diseases by telephone survey: estimates of the frequency and sociodemographic distribution of risk and protective factors for chronic diseases in the capitals of the 26 Brazilian states and the Federal District in 2016. Ministerio da Saude, Secretaria de Vigilancia em Saude, Departamento de Vigilancia de Doenpas e Agravos não Transmissiveis e Promopao da Saude. Brasilia: Ministry of Health, 2017.

BRAZIL. **COFEN Resolution No. 358/2009**. Provides for the Systematization of Nursing Care (SAE) and implementation of the nursing process, in public and private environments where nursing care takes place, and other measures. Brasilia, 2009.

CARPENITO-MOYET, L. J.; GARCEZ, R. M. **Manual of nursing diagnoses.** 13-. ed. Porto Alegre: Artmed, 2011.

CEOLIN, J.; BIASI, L. S. Knowledge of diabetics about the disease and the performance of self-care. Perspectiva, **Erechim**. v. 35, n.129, p. 143156, marpo/2011. Available at: <www.uricer.edu.br/site/pdfs/perspectiva/129_162.pdf.> Accessed on: 20/05/2016.

Diretrizes da Sociedade Brasileira de Diabetes: 2013-2014/Sociedade Brasileira de Diabetes; [organizapao Jose Egidio Paulo de Oliveira, Sergio Vencio]. - Sao Paulo: AC Farmaceutica, 2014. Available at: <https://www.Diabetes.org.br/images/pdf/diretrizes-sbd.pdS.Acesso on: 15/05/2016.

FERREIRA, C. L. R. A.; FERREIRA, M. G. Epidemiological characteristics of diabetic patients in the public health network: analysis based on the HiperDia system. **Arquivos Brasileiros de Endocrinologia e Metabologia,** v. 53, n.1, p.80-86, 2009. Doi:10.1590/S0004-27302009000100012

FERREIRA, D. S. P.; DAHER, D. V.; TEIXEIRA, E. R.; ROCHA, I. J. Repercussão emocional diante do diagnóstico de Diabetes Mellitus tipo 2. **Revista de Enfermagem.** UERJ, Rio de Janeiro, 2013 Jan/Mar. Available at: <www.scielo.br/scielo.php?script=sci_nlinks&pid=S0080...lng=en>. Accessed on: 25/03/2017.

CARVALHO, C. M. A. S.; FERREIRA, A. M. L. **Self-perception of the health of elderly male users of the Planaltina Health Center No. 1. DF**. Universidade Catolica de Brasilia- UCB, 2009. Paper presented to the Universidade Catolica de Brasilia - UCB, for the Degree in Nursing. Supervisor. Prof-. Neuza Moreira de Matos Available at: <https://repositorio.ucb.br/jspui/handle/10869/5001>. Accessed on: 10/02/2018.

GIL, A. C. **Como elaborar projetos de pesquisa.** 4. ed. Sao Paulo: Atlas, 2008.

GIL, G. P.; HADDAD, M. C. L.; GUARIENTE, M. H. D. M. Knowledge about Diabetes Mellitus seen in an interdisciplinary laboratory program at a public university hospital. **Semina: Ciencias Biologicas e da Saude**, Londrina, v. 29, n. 2, jul./dez. 2008. Available at:

<apps.cofen.gov.br/cbcenf/sistemainscricoes/.../I16695.E8.T3408.D4AP.pdf.>
Accessed on: 05/04/2017.

GONQALVES, A. V. F.; RAMOS, M. Z. The different ways of working and
expressing humanization at the Hospital de Clinicas de Porto Alegre. **Revista
Med. Minas Gerais**, 2009. Available at:
<apps.cofen.gov.br/cbcenf/sistemainscricoes/.../I16695.E8.T3408.D4AP.pdf>.
Accessed on: 04/06/2016.

GUYTON, A. C.; HALL, J. E. **HUMAN PHYSIOLOGY.** 12ª edipao. Rio de
Janeiro: Elsevier, 2011.

HORTA, W. A. **Nursing Process.** Sao Paulo: EPU, 1979.

KLAFKE, A.; DUNCAN, B. B.; ROSA, R. S.; MOURA, L.; MALTA, D. C.;
SCHMIDT, M. I. Mortality due to acute complications of diabetes mellitus in
Brazil, 2006-2010. **Epidemiologia e Servipos de Saude**. 2014 Jul-Sep.
Available at: <www.scielo.br/pdf/ress/v23n3/1679-4974-ress-23-03-
00455.pdf>. Accessed on: 22/04/2016.

MALAMAN, L. B. **The process of adherence of diabetic patients to
educational groups as an analyzer of institutional relationships in basic
health units. 2006.** 162 f. Dissertation (Master's) - State University of
Campinas, Postgraduate Program in Collective Health. Available at:
<www.bibliotecadigital.unicamp.br/document/?down=vtls000390950>.
Accessed on: 03/07/2015.

MARASCHIN, J. F.; MURUSSI, N.; WITTER, V.; SILVERIO, S. P.
Classification of Diabetes Mellitus. **Arq. Bras. Cardiologia,** 2010, v. 95, n. 2,
Available at: <www.scielo.br/scielo.php?script=sci_arttext&pid=S0066-
782X2010001200025>. Accessed on: 27/04/2016.

MASCARENHAS, N. B.; PEREIRA, A.; SILVA, R. S.; SILVA, M. G.
Sistematizapao da Assistencia de Enfermagem ao portador de Diabetes
Mellitus e Insuficiencia Renal Cronica. **Revista Brasileira de Enfermagem,**
Jan-Feb; v. 64, n. 1, p. 203-8, Brasilia 2011. Available at:
<http://www.redalyc.org/html/2670/267019462031/>. Accessed on:
15/01/2018.

MENDES, E. V. **The care of chronic conditions in primary health care:** the
imperative of consolidating the family health strategy. Eugenio Vilapa
Mendes. Brasilia: Pan American Health Organization, 2012. 512 p

MINAYO, M. C. S (org.). **Pesquisa social: teoria, metodo e criatividade.** 29. Ed. Petropolis, RJ: Vozes, 2012. (Colepao temas sociais).

MINAYO, M. C. S. **O desafio do conhecimento:** pesquisa qualitativa em saude. 8- ed. Sao Paulo: Hucitec, 2004.

MOREIRA, R. O.; PAPELBAUM, M.; APPOLINARIO, J. C.; MATOS, A. G.; COUTINHO, W. F.; MEIRELLES, R. M. R.; ELLINGER, V. C. M; ZAGURY, L. Diabetes mellitus and depression: a systematic review. **Arquivos Brasileiros de Endocrinologia & Metabologia**, v. 47, n. 1, p. 19-29, 2013. Available at: <http://www.scielo.br/pdf/abem/v47n1/a05v47n1.pdf>. Accessed on: 09/02/2018.

NANDA (North American Nursing Diagnosis Association). **NANDA nursing diagnoses:** definitions and classification 2009-2011. Translated by Regina Machado Garcez. Porto Alegre: Artmed, 2010.

PASQUALOTO, K. R.; ALBERTON, D.; FRIGERI, H. R. Diabetes Mellitus and Complications. **Rev. Biotec. Biodivers**. v. 3, n. 4., November 2012. Available at: <revista.uft.edu.br/index.php/JBB/article/download/385/267>. Accessed on: 28/04/2016.

PERES, D. S.; SANTOS, M. A.; ZANETTI, M. L.; FERRONATO, A. A. Difficulty of diabetic patients to control the disease: feelings and behaviors. **Revista Latino Americana de Enfermagem**, 2007 November-December. Available at: <www.revistas.usp.br/rlae/article/view/16184/17870>. Accessed on: 20/05/2016.

PETERMANN, X. B.; MACHADO, I. S.; PIMENTEL, B. N.; MIOLO, S. B.; MARTINS, L. R.; FEDOSSE, E. Epidemiology and Diabetes Mellitus care practiced in Primary Health Care: a narrative review Saude (Santa Maria). **Revista de Enfermagem de Santa Maria**, v. 41, n.1, p.49-56, 2015. Available at: <https://periodicos.ufsm.br/index.php/revistasaude/article/view/14905>. Accessed on: 14/02/2018.

PONTIERI, F. M.; BACHION, M. M. Beliefs of diabetic patients about nutritional therapy and its influence on adherence to treatment. **Ciencia & Saude Coletiva**, v. 15, n. 1, p.151-160, 2010. Available at: <www.scielo.br/scielo.php?script=sci_arttext&pid=S1413-81232010000100021>. Accessed on: 20/06/2016.

REZENDE, M. F. C. **A case study on the illness experience of type 2**

diabetic users of a Basic Family Health Unit in Araguari-MG. 2010. Dissertation (Professional Master's Degree in Public Health) - Aggeu Magalhaes Research Center, Oswaldo Cruz Foundation, Brasilia, 2010. Available at: <www.cpqam.fiocruz.br/bibpdf/2010rezende-mfc.pdf>. Accessed on: 18/06/2016.

SILVA JUNIOR, F. J. G.; ROCHA, F. C. V.; COSTA, C. S.; CARVALHO, A. B. M. O. **The knowledge of people with Diabetes Mellitus about the complications of the condition.** Graduation work. UNINOVAFAP University Center. PIAUI, 2010. Available at: <apps.cofen.gov.br/cbcenf/sistemainscricoes/.../I16695.E8.T3408.D4AP.pdf>. Accessed on: 22/04/2017.

SMELTZER; S. C; BARE, B. G. Brunner & Suddarth: **Treatise on Medico-Surgical Nursing.** 13- ed. Rio de Janeiro: Guanabara Koogan, 2015. (COLEQAO)

BRAZILIAN DIABETES SOCIETY. Official Positioning No. 2/2015; **Therapeutic Conduct in Type 2 Diabetes:** SBD 2015 Algorithm. Available at: <bibliofarma.com/conduta-terapeutica-no-Diabetes-tipo-2- algoritmo-sbd-2015>. Accessed on: 11/08/2016.

TSCHIEDEL, B. **The History of Diabetes.** Brazilian Society of Endocrinology and Metabology. Sao Paulo: Pfizer, 2006. v.1, p. 34. (A historia do Diabetes, 1). Available at: <www.endocrino.org.br/historia-do- Diabetes>. Accessed on: 05/04/2016.

TANNURE, M. C. PINHEIRO, A. M. **SAE:** Systematization of Nursing Care: a practical guide. 2.ed. Rio de Janeiro: Guanabara Koogan, 2010.

TAVARES, B. C.; BARRETO, F. A.; LODETTI, M. L.; SILVA, D. M. G. V.; LESSMANN, J. C. Resiliences of people with Diabetes Mellitus. **Contexto Texto - Enfermagem.** Florianopolis, v. 20, n. 4, p. 751-757, 2011. Available at: <http://www.scielo.br/pdf/tce/v20n4/14.pdf>. Accessed on: 16/10/2016.

SUMMARY

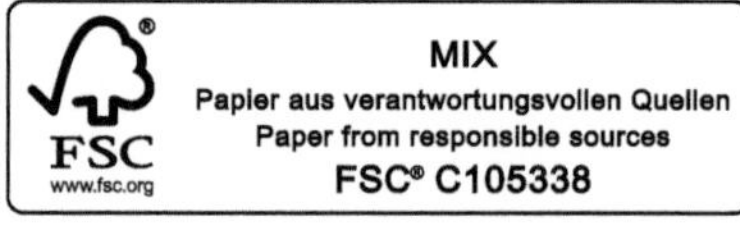

Printed by Books on Demand GmbH, Norderstedt / Germany